A FORMER CHUBBY'S GUIDE TO THE FOREVER FIGURE

A size 20 to a 10

Michelle Mcallister, BSc

ISBN: 978-1-291-85821-1

PublishNation, London

www.publishnation.co.uk

Foreword

Monday mornings are always tough because that's the day when a whole new you starts.......weekend binges always start with "I'll start fresh on Monday!"

This is a guide to fighting the bulge and becoming a better version of you.

The sole purpose of this guide is to ease the woes that come with eating better foods and learning to compromise when stress dictates otherwise. This book is dedicated to those of us who have dealt with the fat jokes, being breathless just walking upstairs, never finding the clothes we like but fit into, being the 'BIG' friend or bridesmaid and countless other comedic situations.

It is also targeted at those of you who could do with learning more about 'fat' people and how overeating isn't always the cause of the problem. Personally I hope that after you read this you drop many pounds, enjoy stress free parties, wear many fab outfits and enjoy life a million times more.

M. Mcallister

CHAPTER 1

AWAKENING

This road has been long and challenging yet the rewards from start to finish are ever present. Losing weight and becoming fitter than I ever imagined has become my biggest achievement to date and I hope that whatever experiences and knowledge I share will help anyone who struggles with weight issues large or small.

As a kid I was tall, lanky and extremely energetic. I played football, cycled and ran everywhere.......your typical active teenager really. I do have a tall slender frame and limbs so was aptly named skeleton or skinny as a kid, not really names that particularly bothered me. I was never focused on my weight as a teenage girl or worried about my looks ....I was far too busy getting muddy or playing with a football. In all honesty my weight did not become a problem for me until I realised I was putting it on and fast!

After sustaining an injury that prevented me from being as active as I once was I started to gain weight rapidly. As most of us may know, the biggest anxiety suppressant has to be food and comfort food can mask a multitude of problems. Eating for comfort can be greatly damaging in many ways but to have no outlet to burn extra food off is even more so. The extra weight becomes the purpose and cause for eating vast amounts of ice cream and crisps. A vicious circle develops and there has to be massive determination to take the all important first step to health by completing the 1st day of improved eating.

Always remember that improved eating is the key to success.......strict diets are a shock to the system and never last long, gradual habit and food choice changes will relieve the monotony of losing excess weight. Most people never tell you how rewarding just completing a day of eating better food really is.....let alone a week or month. Many people see the road ahead as long and challenging but you must remember that your first successful milestone will be close. Simply losing weight or reducing your dress size will give you more motivation than you know. I remember leaping around a changing room because I had squeezed myself into a size 16.......the attendant was virtually a size 8 and couldn't understand my delight. When your born slim, remain slim and stay slim all your life the novelty of looking good is taken for granted.......we voluptuous girls have to work that bit harder to just to get the figure in check before we even start to apply makeup.

Without starting a whole skinny versus heavy battle it is important to remember that unless you have the life experience of a being overweight you can never call yourself an expert in your field.

Being overweight is not only physical but mental too, In order to help someone lose weight it is important to understand their mind set, emotional state and personality. Empathy happens to be my most productive life skill....... I wish I had a pound for every time I have finished the story of a client because they happen to describe something that I have already experienced whilst trying to lose weight.

I have to say here and now that there is nothing worse than a slim girl trying to preach to you about losing weight when she has never faced the issues personally. I've had times when I have walked into classes to teach and I only manage to engage the women participating in weight loss conversation after I tell them that I was once twice my size. I certainly understand that attitude as I would never have taken advice from a skinny girl seriously way back when. I in fact couldn't abide slim girls (no offence meant) but I was prejudice after a few experiences of being called fatty, Bertha, tubby, lard ass and many more truly imaginatively flattering titles........it is amazing how articulate idiots can be.

I think that there may by now have been a few nodding heads in agreement or raised eyebrows. It is always satisfying when someone says exactly what you feel........I've been on both sides. I can't hide my joy when I see a heavy girl stand up for herself because it's taken me years to find my voice.

I think it's time that people start to look past appearances and understand that being heavy is only a temporary barrier in a person's life not the end of it......... I know many fitness instructors who are the fittest around but never gain any real admiration or recognition because they have a heavy appearance.

CHAPTER 2

LEARNING TO IMPROVE ALL AREAS

Becoming a healthier happier person is down to choices and perseverance. Most people who decide to change their appearance tend to rely on quick fixes....... These work short term and yes maybe you'll look amazing at your party, event or wedding but afterwards when your goal had been reached you will simply reward your achievements with a night of heavy booze and hangover scoff, throw that dress in the cupboard and go back to square 1.

I've gone through that scenario many times and after a while it bored me. I realised that a hangover day would be a great release after all the healthy living and believe me I would never deprive anyone of treats and rewards. But rewards come in many different guises so why not think beyond the present and think of rewards that are tangible like new clothes or holidays with the - up until now forbidden bikini packed.

When I decided that I had many parties coming up I started an eating plan that allowed me to stay slim but without the depression of having no nice foods to look forward to....... Having a pizza night or a glass of wine is what life is all about, enjoyment! I always think that celebrities look constantly glum because they probably have to say no to all the nice things in life in order to maintain this whole facade of looking super slim. Half the time celebrities probably have the odd day of bloating and acne anyway so why not treat themselves once in a while. Small periods of feeling good will decrease the stress they place themselves under.

The key is to turn bad habits into good. Many people say that they can't get into good eating habits but if you can fall into the bad ones like junk food you can certainly do the same with sensible foods.

Once I had planned my meals and started to add the foods that I enjoyed it became much easier to develop a habit of sensible eating, staying slim need not be all about rabbit food. There are people who lead busy lives who find planning a nightmare but selecting your meals on an afternoon or day off could be your first major change. Making a large pot of hearty soup or stew and freezing into containers is perfect for having ready meals and saving money by buying large bags of fruits or nuts and dividing into snack size bags is easy.

Being on the go need not mean missing meals – you can always have a snack or piece of fruit with you. I used to think that I would lose more weight if I restricted calories but this led to me eating nothing between lunch and dinner so that I had enough calories in the evening for my treat. Although I lost weight doing this I felt tired in the afternoon and inhaled my dinner because I was famished. Trying to eat small healthy snacks between meals will ensure that your sugar levels never drop and your energy levels will never be compromised. In essence eat breakfast to kick start your metabolism, lunch to maintain energy, a snack to prevent energy dips and after dinner you can enjoy your chosen treat, even if you are counting calories you can still stay satisfied with plenty of whole foods.

If you have a sweet tooth like me and you need a fix there are snacks like wholegrain toast with honey or chocolate spread........it's a compromise that works. There are plenty of sweet treats that will entice your appetite without all the hidden nasties that settle on the waistline.

I've learned to think about how I'll feel if I eat a cupcake when I'm really hungry and how much better I'll feel if I have toast with honey. I've learned now that when I've just completed a heavy exercise session that although my body is like a calorie furnace that it needs the proper carbohydrates and protein to help me feel full and energised.

I am certainly not going to preach about which foods are bad as most people know that there are tasty alternatives and to be honest I am no angel. I enjoy a piece of cake or chocolate bar but I now don't eat as much as I've found great snacks that give me the sweet kick I crave as a chocaholic.

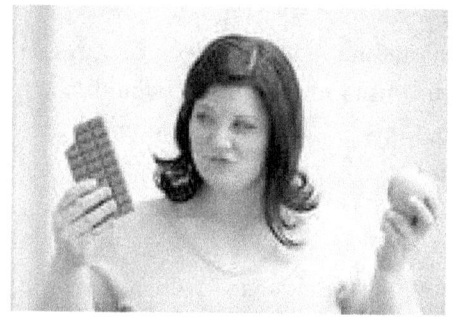

Although I am smaller now I still have the same big appetite I have always had and I never want to change that as I enjoy food and the role it plays in everyday life. The mistake most people make is trying to cut good things out of their lives as oppose to compromising, this inevitably leads to a binge somewhere along the line. I have found that engaging in exercise has helped me to manage the fact that I enjoy a full life with parties and lovely dinners. Exercise has become a saviour for me and becoming a fitness instructor has helped me to change people's attitude to health and sensible eating. I try to finish a session with a good food tip just to encourage participants to think of what they want their post exercise meal to comprise of. Participants like to have a helping hand when deciding when and what to eat after exercising. I've actually met participants who before I spoke to them where going home and eating nothing after classes because they thought that they would lose more weight. Needless to say they retained weight where dehydrated and lost sleep because of it, exercise and good food go hand in hand.

Never underestimate how good you'll feel when you wake up feeling refreshed and hungry for breakfast. Usually you'd probable suffer from confused sugar levels because of what you scoffed the previous night.

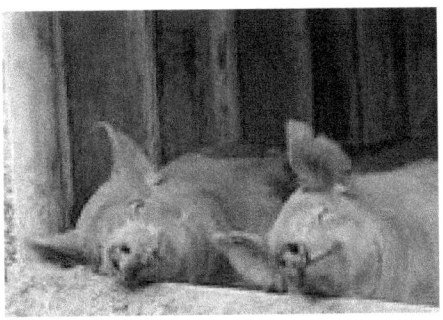

CHAPTER 3

THE MUFFIN TOP REMEDY

Every day on my way to work I would study the various body shapes of the average women I would see making their way to work. I took interest in wardrobe choices and how making small changes could diminish the problem areas that they had unwittingly highlighted.

Having a larger tummy can be a constant nightmare and particularly when it is not in proportion to the body as a whole. Choosing a top that disguises this area will allow you to do so whilst highlighting the areas of your body that please you. Try a top that flows through the midsection. The muffin top effect tends to exist because women and men favour hipsters or ill- fitting jeans, ditch the hipsters until you've lost the midsection fat and invest in a pair of regular jeans that fit you perfectly. This means no overhang and the top needn't have to be floaty - sometimes choosing a larger size of top or darker colour helps to diminish any sign of a large gut.

For the lunches or parties that you attend the perfect dress is out there and not expensive. Darker coloured dresses with light long length light coloured side panels disguise a multitude of sins - these dresses create the illusion of a completely flattering figure so that you feel confident whilst you are on the road to a slimmer appearance.

Take care to choose the best underwear as this'll make or break any outfit. Spilling over a bra, knickers or boxers will demean the effect that you want to present with a flawless outfit choice. An over spilling bra is more often or not the downfall of any smart blouse or fitted dress, this kind of fashion mishap tends to be even more evident with a buxom girl.

Most overweight men will tell you secretly that they have experience of this kind of thing with underwear too so it is important to choose looser fitting boxers on the weight loss road, good fitting shorter length trousers will produce the appearance of longer slimmer legs and these can be jeans or combats whichever makes you feel comfortable.

Perfect the undies until the day when you can step out in dish cloth and feel dazzling......guys!

These tips might sound like common sense but I made many mistakes with my clothes when I was a size 20. Looking back at old photographs now I wonder what made me think that I looked presentable, always try to take a picture when you have an outfit on that you perceive as being risqué. A picture can give you a true reflection of what you really look like, mirrors can be deceiving and it certainly isn't the first time that my mirror at home told me that I looked ok then I venture out in public and see a bag lady in a mirror in town.

The best bet in the long run however is to address the problem head on, weight around the midsection of both genders will almost always be down to poor diet and alcohol consumption. A diet high in saturated fats will place tell-tale signs around the tummy, hips and waist. This is also true of alcohol and in particular beer – a beer belly tells its own story, the beer will absorb straight into the tummy wall causing the pregnancy effect.

Excess fat is the main problem and another causal factor can be excess sugar or fake sweeteners.

CHAPTER 4

BEWARE THE LOW FAT SCANDAL

Diets that profess to low fat are mostly high sugar which is just as bad!

Do not be blinkered when engaging in a new diet, always do your homework and check out all of the foods recommended. If any of the packaging contains low fat but high sugar or sweetener content then ditch it promptly. You have tips for the perfect eating plan in this book and don't ever use the diet word or you are finished before you have begun.

It is a myth that food which is low in fat and sugar has no taste, many natural seasonings are far better on the palette than chemically enhanced e.g. Soya and teriyaki sauce lift any dish adding a meaty kick.

The general public have become used to being brain washed about so called healthy option foods and specific products, the accessibility of these food ranges have made the British public lazy when it comes to eating. It literally takes 20 minutes to oven bake or grill a few chicken breasts in teriyaki sauce whilst cooking bean sprouts, peppers and onions in a pan – you can even have the kettle boiling at the same time for the ginger T that goes perfectly with the meal.

The idea that the work has all been done with convenience foods is tempting for some but the long term harm that can be done should be the warning against them. It is far easier to prepare a quick meal personally and limit the amount of bad additives that are added.

The rainbow effect has become a major selling point in diet products these days. In simple terms this effect is indicative of the advertising and packaging of the product – the bells, whistles and false images that draw the consumer in. Aspiring to look like the guy or girl in the advert is the main selling point but surely health is as important as physical appearance and both can be achieved with a natural eating plan. The chemicals in certain foods leave the consumer craving more which probably shouldn't be a good reason for buying more – there is a difference between eating food because of enjoyment and eating because your addicted to it and need it. A sugar or sweetener high will last temporarily then leave you with the slump and need for another hit whereas a natural sugar found in honey or peanut butter will satisfy you for hours.

A diet high in sweeteners or added sugar will lead to fat storage unless the recipient is working out like a demon daily.

These are not meant as scare tactics but as general information to arm yourself with when you choose foods, sometimes a little of what you fancy does you good so try honey treats or natural sugars.

Eating natural foods will not break the bank like the old days as these foods are more accessible at reasonable prices. Use the bulk option for the power to control portion size. Purchase an affordable cook book that offers education in steaming foods, portion control, natural alternatives and snack ideas.

CHAPTER 5

EXERCISE CAN BE YOUR SAVIOUR

Not only will exercise help you to stay slim and maintain a really enjoyable lifestyle but it also will surprise you big time...... exercise will be your new habit.

I found that when I got into exercising that it became my new obsession. I tend to develop habits quickly and it was good to replace my bad eating habits with good training habits. There have been people in the past who have warned against the dangers of over exercising and even described it as a "disorder". Are athletes at risk of an exercise disorder? After all they train for fair amounts daily and become passionate about their sport. As long as you are aware of your increased fuel intake and post session rest the risk of disorder should never be an issue. I was training every day when I first started training again and I felt energised every morning. I made sure that my water intake was adequate and I enjoyed a fantastic diet with my treats also. When I started teaching I actually had to increase my food intake as I noticed a dramatic change in my weight .... Ironic since I had been trying years to do something that happened almost overnight with an increased exercise regime.

When I tell clients that everything falls into place when they eat sensibly and exercise I really speak the truth and I'm living proof. I can't remember a time that my life was so organised and happy. For me when I'm eating the right foods and getting my exercise done I feel more efficient in work endeavours, I enjoy my social life and sleep like a baby.

There are many forms of exercise to engage in and everyone should have some type of exercise to enjoy. As long as you are getting warm, sweaty, using your lungs and feeling an endorphin release you should be burning calories. For most people it is about the waistline and eating good whole foods will help you reduce the tummy bulge.

I have exercised now for years since I lost my 4 stone excess and I do believe that without exercise I would have struggled. Not everyone has time to devote to exercise sessions but a 30 minute burst has made the difference to a great deal of my client's lives. I started tailoring 30 minute boot camp sessions to their and my needs and it worked with dramatic results.

Around the time I became involved in my new choice of training I had gained 7 pounds of holiday weight. Most people hadn't noticed but I did and especially when I was running, it is amazing the difference 7 pounds can seem when you measure it in blocks of cheese or bags of sugar.

As I say I am a creature of habit and I do make the mistake of over doing something too much when I need to vary my workouts. With me its running, I enjoy running and can sometimes get bogged down improving my running time when I should really be adapting and adding to my workout variety. When I realised that the running was not helping me shift my excess weight I decided to participate in my client's calorie bursting sessions.

It is important here to remind you that exercise variety is the key to preventing boredom and to improve weight management. If you think of stimulating your body like stimulating your mind the idea makes sense. No person reads the same page of a book over and over, this would bore you and provide no mental stimulation.......you'd become stagnant. Your body becomes accustomed to the same movements and patterns therefore you need to challenge and vary everything that you do. If you think about completing a class or session that was new and different you'll know that you work harder and become more alert, it is also gratifying when you are successful in overcoming new exercise concepts.

I remember chatting to clients when they had come to me for advice and asking about their history up until our point of contact. Around 8 out of 10 clients had said that they became bored with their previous trainers workouts because they became easy or repetitive. It is essential for any trainer to realise that when clients become fitter and more confident that the content of their training schedule should reflect this. Failing to recognise that clients have improved stamina, agility, strength and power is unacceptable and can stunt any results in terms of weight loss and muscle conditioning. I will never have my clients try any type of exercise or movements that I haven't tried myself. I like my classes and sessions to be active and I always participate 100% in everything I teach – I leave my sessions looking like I've been dragged through a hedge but when you feel energised the effort you put in shows.

The 30 minute sessions I have tailored to clients with busy lives, children, high pressure jobs etc have been really successful. Basically the more effort you put in the better results will be and because people know that it is a short period of effort they then tend to go for it. The results are really impressive, I used myself and my friends as guinea pigs when I designed the sessions and we all dropped an average of 8 pounds in the first 2 weeks.

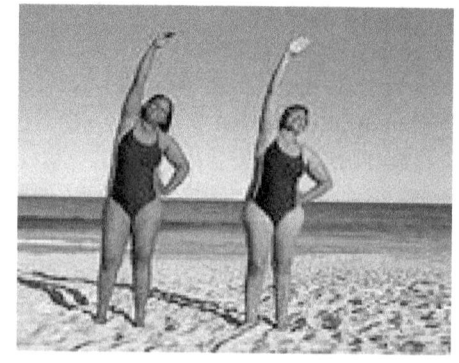

The sessions where 3-4 days weekly at various times and reps of specific exercises that would improve strength, agility, bone density and heart\lung strength. Ultimately these sessions would inspire my clients to reach target weights and fitness goals sooner than they ever imagined.

CHAPTER 6

YOYO DIETING

I feel like I've become something of an expert when it comes to diets and the feelings that they conjure up. To me diet means deprivation, it is something that describes a person's daily food intake and not what they should become enslaved to. I always think that 'diet' like 'fat' has had its true meaning overhauled and a new stigmatic meaning applied....fat is not what we are it is what we carry and it is not a dirty word either........good fats are our friend. Ignorance has a big part to play in the overuse of both words and I can justify to that after being called fat for many years.

Sometimes with the yoyo dieter it takes something small or uneventful to make them realise that their behaviour is calculated. Have you ever had a day where you say to someone "I've just realised I haven't eaten any garbage Today", well I have. It seems to me that you can go a whole week without eating your favourite junk food and not even think about it. This is the key to eating better foods ....don't think so much about it. It's when you think that you need junk food that you crave it. If you try new foods that you like you might even find that you'll replace your old foods with the new ones, I remember having an attack of the munchies 1 day and instead of inhaling some chocolate I had some lovely cereal – it was actually bran and I enjoyed it so much that I started to use it for my snack as oppose to the kitkat I had become accustomed to having....... There goes that habit again!

When I looked at my eating patterns since I had first started trying to lose weight I noticed that I had been yoyo dieting for a long time. Hine sight allows insightfulness after the event but at the time I thought that I would lose weight, many people do.

I would always start my diet on the Monday get depressed and by Tuesday evening would give in and promise myself that I would DEFINITELY do it the following week. Well the weekend would come and I simply had to have pizza and wine.......I don't know anyone who would aim to start a diet on a weekend day, it's a ludicrous suggestion for a dieter to consider. I used to eat and be merry on the Saturday and Sunday and promise myself that when Monday came I would be determined to start my revolution.

Thinking and doing are completely different things and when a person is fully committed to losing excess weight they will do it. I just had several dry runs but made it eventually and wow what a week that was! Once I knew that I wasn't on a "diet" but better eating kick I became successful for the first time at actually losing weight.

Yoyo dieting can be the easiest trap to fall into and many people try various different diets because of the fabulous results they promise to deliver. No one ever tells you that the celebrities who follow these diets have help along the way and certainly don't live the average lifestyle. It's a shame that most women pin their hopes on the latest diet available........common sense would tell you that your body needs more than a bowl of cabbage soup or a glass of honey and chilli! But that is the pull that losing weight has and particularly with females.

I know that men struggle with weight and that they can also sometimes become emotional eaters but the pressure on women to look as good as those in the public eye is tremendous and extremely unfair. No average woman has a private PT, house gym, dress designer or personal chef so they rely on the only thing that resembles their favourite role model...... a fad diet. I speak from experience and can reveal that we can lose weight with better resources and relish the results more.

Losing weight will be the inevitable result for you when you feel ready and have complete power of the choices you make. Being shamed, forced or pressured into weight loss by everyone else in your circle whether that be family, friends or partners will end with an argument, dent in your ice cream stash and you back at square one.

Think easy! If you perceive this as easy it'll make things easier and personal praise will keep you striving toward your ultimate goal.

The starting point on this road is a plan of action – when you feel that you are slipping do one of these things:-
1. STRESS FREE BAKING OR MEAL PLANNING
2. EXERCISE BURSTS – EVEN 5 MINUTES IS ENOUGH
3. MOTIVATIONAL FILMS – ROCKY, OR ANYTHING WITH TRAINING MONTAGUES
4. DANCE – STICK ON PINK IN CONCERT OR YOUR FAVOURITE STAR AND DANCE ALONG
5. WASH THE CAR OR GET THE DRIVEWAY IN ORDER
6. CALL A FRIEND FOR A NIGHT OUT WITH LOADS OF DANCING
7. GET YOUR PARTNER TO CHASE YOU AROUND THE PARK NEAR YOU
8. TAKE THE KIDS TO THE NEAREST PLAY AREA OR SWING PARK AND HAVE A GO

Sometimes simple actions in life can be the catalyst for a week full of motivation, the next time that you feel drained get your ipod bouncing with the kind of music that you never thought you would be dancing to. Music and film empower people with the energy they never thought imaginable so get moving.

CHAPTER 7

EMOTIONAL EATERS

I can't state this as a Fact but from my personal experience of clients stories, people I know and my knowledge of psychology I understand that women tend to eat for comfort whereas men see food as fuel. That is for around 60% of the male's life as the other 40% will probably be spent having comfort food as he engages in a new relationship. You all know what it's like when you start dating someone the eating out and cosy takeaways become a feature of your lifestyle.

The difference between men and women is that most women have dieted in order to attract that man and so gain the weight they have lost whilst dating him whilst men simply gain a few pounds during dating and can lose it easily, they don't see this as a battle, they will just hit the gym a few times.

Most females tend to see weight gain as a battle and I do say most because there are the exceptions. I only wish that we could have the mind set of most men......"it's just a few pounds I'll burn it off at gym", that is really what it is after all. Most women, and I speak personally too when I state that "I need to lose about a stone" when really it's a couple of pounds.

That is all part of the female's dramatic charm but it does us no favours when we analyze the way we look because we never see what other people do.

I tend to use food as a reward or as an essential part of my telly experience. I know that some people reward themselves with clothes, music and socialising but I used to buy wine or chocolates. I can remember planning out my night of goodies if I was having a quiet Saturday night in, from my dinner to my ice cream I almost made a list of the order. I remember that my Wednesday sex and the city night used to be a 6 pack of crisps and litre tub of ice cream......that was before the weekend had come ....and I used to wonder why I was so big.

When I lost my weight I used to worry about parties and nights out and how I would resist the temptation of the blow outs I had before. This can be quite tough and lead to the calling off of several good nights. Learning to understand when you are satisfied and have had enough is essential. There is a feeling of fulfilment that occurs probably around the main course of a meal that I often missed or ignored, I am fine now with 1 glass of wine and a pasta main whereas before I seen it as my duty to have all courses and a bottle of wine. I think that if I didn't have a dessert or starter that I felt I was cheating myself and not embracing the enjoyment of eating out.

My brain writes cheques my tummy can't cash and when I started listening to my tummy I became better at stopping when I was full. Even when you are full a colourful dessert can usually tip you over the edge. Rationalising how you'll feel if you eat that dessert works and even recollecting past experiences when overeating has made you feel awful will act as a deterrent.

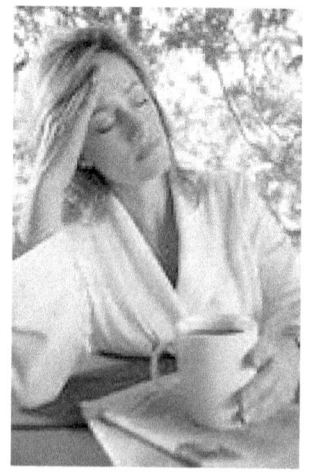

I always find that the morning after feeling also helps me rationalize if I need another cake or glass of wine, there is no crappier feeling than the morning after a binge and that is ammunition enough against ever doing it.

CHAPTER 8

CELEBRITY FADS AND HARMFUL DIETS

It has become apparent that in this day and age most women aspire to the typical celebrity fad diet - this should never be an option unless the celebrity practises a regime of safe eating patterns. Celebrities who decide to follow eating plans that consist of one, little or no foods may look good on the outside but they will be creating untold damage on the internal organs resulting in premature internal aging.

A complete eating plan should consist of meals and snacks that incorporate all food groups. These groups will provide the essential vitamins, minerals and nutrients needed for the human body to self-cleanse, replenish, function and operate properly daily with or without exercise.

The human body is after all a machine that requires necessary fuel, feeding an adult 500 calories daily as oppose to the recommended 2000 or 2500 will lead to that individual hitting a very large wall.

Calorie restriction will ultimately lead to fat storage – the brain hits the red button when a reduction in calories occurs. Add in exercise and the panic button will be ringing! - the higher the calories in proper quality nutritious foods the more efficient the body becomes and the better it is equipped to burn unwanted fat faster.

Most people like to track the calories they consume in order to lose weight with the input/output method. This is effective however most tend to complain about where the weight drops from with the gut being the last place. Although you can't spot shift fat it is a good idea to try foods that exist in low GI eating. If you consume nutritious natural foods sensibly you will not feel the need to count calories as you will see the weight shift. Low GI foods will be eaten in moderation simply because they keep people fuller for longer, because these foods stabilise sugar levels the need to overeat does not occur and fat storage reduces. Less bad fats mean that the gut becomes an area where fat reduces – it is simply a diet of bad fats that leave this area thicker.

If calorie counting is your preferred choice then remember to stick with 2000 calories whilst you exercise and lose the unwanted weight. As soon as you are at a healthy weight it is important to up the calorific intake to 2500 calories daily – the extra 500 will support your daily exercise routines. Now if you train particularly fiercely then it is important to realise that a hefty boot camp, spin combat or body attack session can leave you with a 700 calorific burn so use the extra 200 calories wisely with an extra lean chicken fillet at dinner or perhaps an evening bowl of porridge when the hunger pangs usually show up. After a workout simply think of what you have used, depleted, exhausted and drained – replenish fuel and water stores effectively then get some rest.

CHAPTER 8

THE TIME IS NOW

Age should never become an issue when thinking of losing weight, people can achieve anything at any age. I am far fitter in my late thirties than I ever was in my twenties. Most of my clients are in their forties or above and the best advert for my work that I could hope for. I have 1 client in particular who had never been near a gym in her life but had overcome smoking to join the gym in the same day. Needless to say she lost weight and has taken part in my lung bursting, flat out fat burning sessions for years. The sessions are great for her motivation as every single person involved has faced similar struggles to hers, I don't entertain anyone who isn't part of the group. The key to all of us losing weight is to work together – even when I teach a class there is an unspoken respect among the group as we can appreciate how hard the next person works. When I teach these sessions I get to feel like a warrior for 45 minutes as do the participants, I think that exercise has taken on the role of escapism in the average person's life. It's cliché but empowerment is a great motivational tool and has replaced any urges I have for junk food or wine.

Some members of the group have experienced injury during workouts but have come back stronger and this serves as good motivation for the others. An injury is merely a temporary setback with alternative workouts becoming readily available. I have enjoyed seeing clients become delighted that they have trimmed their bingo wings as a result of an alternative session. One lady had always had major upper body issues as a result of losing a great deal of weight she had experienced some skin sagging. When she injured her ankle I created an upper body workout that left her with ripped arms and strong abdominals, not bad for a forty eight year old.

In my experience I have met many doubters who are sure that they can never lose weight or improve general fitness with the help of some activity. The best part of my job is proving them wrong and gaining their trust. I know through personal experience the doubts or concerns they may harbour and empathy can be a great tool in reassuring them.

So, what if you can't exercise?

There are times when people simply can't exercise and I want there to be an answer for everyone. A percentage of the population go past the point where they can exercise safely or comfortably because of the strain that excess weight has placed on their body. Joint pain or difficulty breathing can be barriers to exercise and sometimes taking things gradually works more effectively. This is the point where an eating plan can kick start weight reduction until exercise can be an option, or even if exercise is not an option.

A low GI eating plan is extremely useful in stabilising sugar levels and can help diabetics and the obese regulate their levels in order to prevent weight gain. This is a good start and in order to reduce weight the "fuller for longer" approach is necessary. Reducing the high sugar foods you have daily and incorporating whole grains ensure that you never feel the need to snack. Your body will become more efficient when processing good foods and you'll actually burn unwanted fat. This eating plan can accommodate those with a savoury craving or sweet tooth with natural foods such as honey or peanut butter.

It can be easy to become disheartened when you are not able to exercise but this eating plan is miraculous. For those who have become accustomed to exercise there is one subject that is a scary prospect to behold ....INJURY. Like me most people have the philosophy that they can have those guilty pleasures as long as they counteract them with FAT BURNING......what if you can't fat burn though?

I highlight those words because of the significance they hold in the world of us compromisers. It makes sense to those of us who have acquired the taste for chocolate to make a compromise instead of cutting out of our lives altogether...... where's the fun in that? Remember the faces of those who depress themselves by cutting out every little pleasure in life to stay ultra slim. When exercise becomes 1 of the excuses, eh I mean tools (gym bunny joke) that you use to enjoy a full life it can be a disruptive inconvenience daily when you can't burn off excess calories. The mental uplifting that comes with blasting pumping music in a class or your ipod whilst you jump, run and sweat cannot be replaced and in some cases can lead to depression.

Most people who have never exercised to music cannot fully appreciate how much better a person feels after a session – everything just seems better and the bonus of calories burned makes it worthwhile ....Rocky soundtrack music tends to work. I feel that I can speak empathetically about injury as I have gone through a hideous knee injury that halted my exercise regime in its tracks. I basically could not do the classes or personal fat burning sessions that I had taken for granted and I was floored.

After feeling sorry for myself and comfort eating for a bit I realised that I could compromise and tailor a programme to my needs, this experience would serve as a great learning curve and inspiration for my clients and their exercise needs. I was unable to do any impact work and so spent time in the local swimming pool where I learned to strengthen my whole body and maintain cardiovascular strength.....there was no way I was about to lose the fitness levels that I had built over years and had become known for. A big part of dealing with an injury is realising that you are not invincible and are unable (for that period only) to perform the exercises that you had before.

The pool work served as a great way to burn fat and I taught myself some new exercise techniques that would be invaluable with clients for session variety. I scrutinised the upper body work sessions I had designed before and created many new short burst programmes that would help me enjoy this genre again. I loathed doing any strength work but always did as I knew it was an essential part of my work. Learning new exercise patterns was a good tonic in my recovery, my clients also benefited as they knew that injury would certainly not prevent me or them from exercising in the event of an injury .... I led by example as always.

Depression can still become an unwelcome factor even if you do find a way to exercise. You have time to think and realise that you take your body for granted. For some people it takes longer to overcome and they do need extra help but that is in no way a sign of weakness, this simply means that finding your way back is even more satisfying.

During these times it often helps to listen to the music that motivates you or even to write about your feelings. This sounds airy fairy but it often becomes therapeutic and can inevitably help others who face injury, I hope this does.

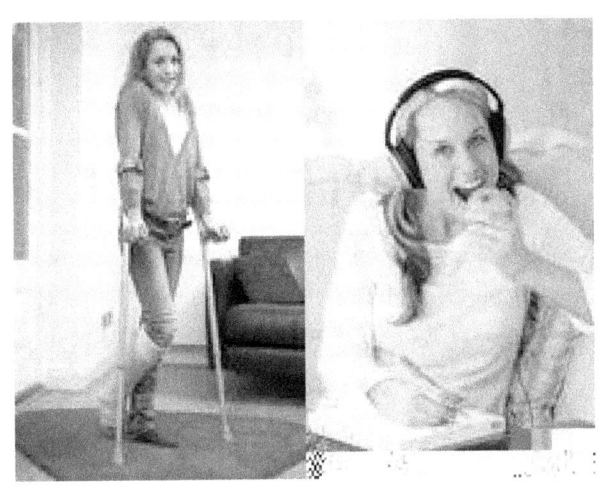

INJURY CAN BE POSITIVE!

CHAPTER 9

LOW GI TIPS AND CHOICES

Low GI foods keep you satisfied for longer which means that eating every 4 hours will be something that becomes habitual to your everyday routine. If however you do become peckish there are many snack choices available.

DRINKS WITH EVERY MEAL
1. WATER
2. HOT WATER WITH LEMON
3. GREEN OR GINGER TEA
4. MINT TEA OR CAMMOMILE FOR DIGESTION
5. PURE UNSWEETENED CRANBERRY OR ORANGE JUICE

BREAKFAST
1. Wholegrain cereals & berries/citrus fruits (bananas can play havoc with sugar levels)
2. Porridge with cinnamon, honey, salt, nuts or low sugar   jam
3. Wholegrain or Burgen toast with honey or peanut butter
4. Toast with eggs scrambled or poached
5. Fruits blended with yoghurt or milk (5 fruits)
6. Fruit salad with natural yoghurt and honey or grated   dark chocolate (4 squares)
7. Beans with low sugar sauce on wholegrain toast
8. Grilled, trimmed bacon with grilled tomato
9. Wholegrain wraps with eggs or trimmed bacon
10. Wholegrain pancakes with fresh berries

Wholegrain is an easier choice because it is widely available in supermarkets.

LUNCH

1. Hearty vegetable or tomato soup with wholegrain crackers
2. Pan fried or grilled chicken with light sauce and brown noodles
3. Sweet potato with seared beef or turkey
4. Toast with eggs and feta or helium cheese
5. White wine or chicken stock with natural yoghurt for carbonara or chicken
6. Beef stock and blended beans can be great thick sauce
7. Feta cheese with wine or stock provides great cheese sauce
8. Low sugar coconut milk with chicken stock and curry powder makes good thick sauce

DINNER DELIGHTS

1. Hearty venison stew in vegetable stock with sweet potato and carrot
2. Sweet potato wedges in extra virgin olive oil with char grilled chicken and sauce
3. Grilled fish on a bed of couscous with sauce choice and dill garnish
4. Brown noodles tossed in light sauce with chicken slices and stir fry vegetables
5. Brown pasta in garlic tomato sauce with sliced or shredded grilled turkey
6. Stir fry cod pieces in peanut butter sauce with julienne carrots and sweet peas.
7. Seafood selection in light dressing (low sugar) with grated carrot coleslaw (Grate carrot and onion or cabbage and toss in light thousand island dressing – garnish with herbs or ground nuts).Pouring warm pasta sauce over a salad or baked sweet potato can beef it up a little

SNACKS AND BETWEEN MEAL FILLERS

If you are not full between meals and feel the need for a small snack to maintain energy levels try to resist any foods that elevate sugar levels unnecessarily. The feeler of hunger will never be satisfied with sugar, you will only crave more so try to compromise with natural sugars if you must have something sweet.

Carrots have a low GI score and can be sliced to dip into peanut butter which also has a low score. Nuts in general will fulfil you and provide protein also so why not have some crushed nuts in yoghurt or over fruit. I like to have a small bowl of bran or wholegrain based cereals to curb hunger in the afternoon – a ready-made mini meal.

Just remember that a snack is simply something that keeps your engine ticking over until your next meal so small packs of fruits and nuts can be eaten on the go.

Snack choices are fruitful so the need for chocolate bars will become a thing of the past.

1. Fill a small bags with raisins or sultanas and broken walnuts or brazil nuts
2. Wholegrain snacks like crackers or biscuits can be bought in snack size packs
3. Bananas, apples, Clementine oranges, kiwis, plums, nectarines and grapes all provide natural sugars but remember to vary choices
4. 1 single slice of Burgen bread with low fat spread can be just enough with a cup T
5. If you really must have chocolate of some description try a few Jaffa cakes and if dark chocolate won't suffice try a Reece's peanut butter cup

Tips for tasty dishes

1. Sauces can be adapted to reduce added fat and sugar – try boiling tomatoes and adding mushrooms, onions, peppers and garlic or even softening some low fat cheese spread with some crushed garlic and lean chopped grilled bacon then pouring over couscous. It's amazing how good things can taste with proper seasoning.

2. Soya sauce adds flavour and oomph to any dish but especially chilli wholegrain noodles or rice

3. Garlic adds to any dish from a warm salad to a bowl of tomato soup

4. Herbs like chives can be added to natural yoghurt or mayo to create a new dressing or dip

5. Sesame or extra virgin olive oil can provide tasty healthier options for dressing ingredients

6. Oregano chopped over light soft cheese and warm tomatoes creates an indulgent but healthy snack

7. Lemon juice can be warmed and mixed with chopped red chilli to dress cod, hake, sardine, tuna or even salmon

8. Overall there are choices that can make a significant difference to how you keep the eating plan interesting and successful. Try looking at low GI websites and books to collect the menus and food choices that you need for variety and your cooking skills will benefit also. There are many diets out there that promise weight loss but most tend to suggest foods that are pre packed, high in sugar and low in fat. Any pre packed foods that do not clearly state what ingredients are used should be avoided. You will benefit from dismissing pre packed foods that produce flavour by over salting or adding hideous amounts of sugar.

Low fat is a term that has been over used since the diet fad started and people fall for it every time. Low fat meals usually have more sugar and this is the easiest way to heighten sugar levels and subsequently hold onto fat. The good fats are beneficial in moderation as are the omega 3 and 6 fats – found in nuts and oily fish. Women benefit greatly from omega 6 and you'll also save yourselves a fortune in cod liver oil capsules if you include regular portions of fish and nuts in your eating plans.

It is fun when you can create dishes from the low GI food choices that are available – my best ever discovery was the frittata and I was able to use the left over sliced vegetables from the night before. Everyone always has eggs in the fridge and the addition of onions, peppers, mushrooms and tomatoes will fill the meal out along with some crumbled feta for substance.

CHAPTER 10

OVERCOMING THE BARRIERS THAT LEAD TO BREAKING THE CYCLE

Everyone has been there at some point, the eating plan is going well and you are satisfied until the party or dinner invitation comes up. This section will give the support you need to get through the pressures of over eating and drinking at events.

Peer pressure is a strong ingredient to add to the mix and when you have friends or partners who do not need to stick to your plan or who don't understand why you can't consume as much as they do then a helping hand is useful.

Arm yourself with a strong attitude, if telling yourself that you'll ultimately look and feel better than all the friends who mock your eating plan then go for it.......who are you hurting by using this as motivation? Tell yourself that you'll feel and look fresher the next day when others have hangover effects and it works every time. Enjoying a meal or few drinks is really all you need , always think of how you feel when you order that extra dish or drink that you don't really want......you never enjoy it and more often than not it's that one indulgence that leads to the yucky feeling next morning.

Gaining strong motivation is a skill that is built over years of many bad food or drink experiences. Most people go overboard with perhaps a dessert or extra glass of wine and pay the price psychologically but if you never experience these events you'll have nothing to use as tangible motivation.

Eating out can be a lovely experience as oppose to the daunting task that people who diet perceive it to be. Just remember that the people who mock probably have their own insecurities. I always had people taunt me during Saturday night parties about getting up on the Sunday to workout but as they spent their Sunday feeling dehydrated, exhausted, hungry for junk and depressed I had already exercised and felt fresh as a daisy on my way to a fun day out.

Forget about what other people say, ultimately you are the person who will always have the clothes you like as oppose to the only size that fits. You are the person who will plan fun weekends for you and your family and you will even wake up on Monday mornings feeling refreshed – good eating and hydration influence all areas of life from brain function to digestive system to energy levels. Red bull and caffeine diminish as you eat better when you retrieve the nutrients your body needs from natural sources.

It is surprising how your mind-set changes when you start to engage in new routines and you'll change without even realising it. Sometimes being a creature of habit can be a positive thing when you start any lifestyle change because after a few days you'll become accustomed to specific foods and eating regularly, arranging eating times will become part of your everyday duties, much like picking out clothes or shoes.

Use ant tool that helps you along the way whether that be a food diary or wall chart as long as you can keep track of how well your doing or of any food patterns that may arise – you want to keep all things in moderation so try not over indulge in any particular foods or exercise because inevitably you'll tire of it ,this journey will enable you to try things you never even thought of .You will broaden your horizons and meet people who are in exactly the same position as you are.

CHAPTER 11

MOTIVATION TOOLS

1. Curb false hunger by eating a good meal before nights out and drink water or green T
2. Plan a day out for the day after so that you commit to drinking sensibly
3. Drink water between glasses of wine or keep some natural sugar sources in your handbag such as a few grapes or sesame snaps
4. Keep a good breakfast aside for the day after to prevent breakfast snacking or junk like fried eggs or bacon
5. State to people from the get go that you have plans the next day and will moderate your alcohol intake but are up for a good night
6. Try to explain to the group how good you feel when you follow your fit rules and organise a day or fun that involves you all
7. Always reinforce how good you look when you have lost weight and maybe your attitude will inspire others
8. Dance as much as you can and when you are thirsty order water before you sip wine – never drink alcohol for thirst it has the opposite effect
9. Tell non- believers that their favourite hobby of dancing is the perfect exercise and even throw in the one about sex too that should convince them
10. Try to organise the crowd so that there are a few gym goers among you – often the talk will steer towards the benefits of exercise

11. Study the venues that offer healthy options or organise venues that will accommodate you and your eating arrangements so that you can order whatever you want

12. It is a misconception that red wine has less sugar then white and if you want to make a better choice drink sparkling wine, you'll also feel fuller with the bubbles

13. Often diet drinks contain more sugar so study the best choices if you enjoy spirits – sometimes pure fruit juice is best as it contains natural sugars

14. When arriving home after a few drinks consume water, natural sugar (found in spoonful of honey) or fruit bar and preferably a small glass of milk

15. Once you've consumed your damage control try to get as much sleep as possible – it helps in all areas to and your Sunday will be brighter if you are.

16. Always ensure that your hydrated before, during and after exercise or nights out so drink before, sip during and drink plenty after to replenish what you have depleted

17. If you have days out planned with friends always work out when and where you'll be eating, it's easy and fun to prepare a picnic or suggest the new sushi place for you all.

18. If you have the urge for a lovely baked treat try having a go yourself, wholegrain or brown flour are great for cakes but so are ground almonds. Ground almonds are as substantial as flour but provide better nutritional value and fruit juice or honey can be used as alternative 'natural' sweeteners along with good quality chocolate for toppings

19. Get online and check out the many healthy recipes you can choose for dinner parties, buffets, picnics and general meal planning. There are also loads of healthy option cook books to choose from so if your loved ones are stuck for Birthday present ideas for you try dropping a few hints.

CHAPTER 12

REFRESH THE EXERCISE ROUTINE

One thing that has become common between the men and women who take steps to improve their daily food intake and exercise quota is the need to keep everything fresh and motivated. Exercise is bound to be chore like if it never progresses to a higher level or different genre, for anyone embarking upon a radical new activity plan the first few weeks will be a challenge but the success in short term time limits will spark a new thirst for sweat that will outweigh any fatigue. Within one month to six weeks there will be a greater need for natural progressions to more difficult techniques and session arrangements. At this particular point it is important to have decided upon the next step and specific areas in the physique that require extra help.

Whatever the workout may be it is necessary that interval training become an integral part of any programme – this type of training not only strengthens the CV system far more effectively than say simple monotonous jogging but it burns fat like a furnace. Always think of the health benefits and improving your bone density before you consider the fat burning aspect – health should always be your priority. This training will allow you to become more explosive than you could imagine, achieving fitness goals you thought unreachable and in the process blowing your self-confidence high, this is the type of cycle that will enhance your whole approach to exercise and in turn you will burn fat and lose weight in a healthy way. At this point your capabilities will outweigh any doubt you harbour.

The most seasoned exercisers follow the premise of progression in order to challenge themselves and keep sessions interesting. Spontaneity is the key to fitness success so keep a notebook of strategies as you further your knowledge of effective exercises. Most instructors relay a depth of information during classes in order to keep participants safe and motivated. If you are not learning more about progressions, alternative classes, tougher techniques and goal setting then find your vice and ask. When I teach I ensure that as I perform exercises I repeat safety instruction whilst sensitively correcting any potential injury risks – often the biggest cause of injury is poor technique! Also I explain which muscle groups are being utilised and how effective each exercise Is– highlighting which muscle is being loaded will help educate people and inform those too embarrassed to ask, participants will give 110% if they feel assured in their ability and that they are executing the move safely! Reinforcing information in sessions is the best tool for safety and imagery can also help people pick up difficult moves – a simple image helped me teach an upper cut to many in my class. Once in the gym I was approached by a lady who had been experiencing jarring hip pain and she had recently started a class where she was kicking, on inspecting I had noticed that she failed to turn her heel and shift her weight so she was effectively attempting to turn her leg without moving her foot hence the hip load. All this women needed was a step by step picture of how she would perform the kick in slow motion and an image of the target in front instead of to the side, once she took around five minutes to do this she realised her mistake and over time eradicated the hip jarring.

Taking the time to incorporate direction into all the yells and shouts of encouragement pays dividends not only for me as an instructor but for the participants. I felt assured that my class team always left sessions with understanding of the components and the relevance of them. I wanted them to understand why I had tailored the sessions to their particular needs and what they would achieve from them-I wanted them to feel confident that they could plan personal sessions. My participants knew more about nutrition and hydration in comparison to the training they engaged in and reported significant improvements in their performances and recoveries. To offer informed instruction in classes is to save exercisers from unnecessary injury and empower them to explore the exercise world in a safe environment. Online classes are useful but there is never an observer to pick up on the small mistakes so in the long run it is wise to attend a few classes and learn as much as you can before you attempt your own session.

On the odd occasion that I've had a spare hour I would usually prepare a short concise handout for my participants to take home and study- perhaps an outline of the most effective moves in a class or suggestions of what to eat and drink when arriving home. An exercise class can be a daunting prospect for new comers so a friendly chat before the class to gain some background on the people will help them feel included and allow the instructor to gage their strengths.

If you feel confident enough to pursue a workout alone or you simply have no time and have to work out whenever you can try these sessions- there really is no EXCUSE!

CHAPTER 13

QUICK AND EASY WORKOUTS

WHERE TO START – NEWCOMER WORKOUT
Start slowly until you build up in all areas from strength to confidence.

30 MINUTE SESSIONS TWICE WEEKLY
With these sessions you should include jogs, planks, light weights and stretches. There are loads of ideas available in this book and if you can make every session different then you'll work twice as hard. Through time you can increase workouts to 4 times weekly and 45 minutes also.

SUGGESTIONS
20 minutes short intervals of 2 minute jog\2 minute light runs
10 minutes total body work with kettle bell or free weights –research reputable sites for effective safe exercise ideas
10 minutes core work, the core supports every move you make in daily life so it makes sense to strengthen the area. Find appropriate exercises that will isolate the core and strengthen the lower back too – if you eat properly and follow the fitness rules your abs will shine and without all the dangerous crunches.
5 minutes stretch and wind down-research the most effective stretches and when confident attempt multi muscle group stretches, these save time and can help improve balance.

PROGRESS to the intermediate workout within six weeks although your body will let you know when your next challenge should come.

INTERMEDIATE WORKOUT

This workout is also perfect for the people who have been doing the same old exercise routine for years.

55 minute sessions twice weekly
30 minute boot camp twice weekly-if possible perform these sessions at differing times of the week day.
35 minute swim with easy intervals

When training outdoors, never forget that outdoor climates can result in higher fat burning potential-always keep the body guessing by mixing up all elements of the workout when you can.

55 minutes should include:-
25 minutes sprint/run intervals 2/4 minutes each and if this seems easy simply lower the recovery time from 4 to 2 minutes. Uphill or wind sprints will enhance core strength-never let weather be a deciding factor in your workout!

20 minutes of compound exercises with kettle bell-get the whole body working as a complete unit and double the intensity with a Turkish get up or swing sequence-you could even surprise yourself with an impromptu get up challenge and see how many you can complete in 5 minutes.

10 minutes dedication to stretches and breathing practise-this will help when weight training and will teach you how to breathe properly as you execute lifts. Postural care websites that are reliable will outline the basis for posture, correct breathing patterns in relation to lifting and how to use the diaphragm effectively.

EXPERIENCED EXERCISER WORKOUT

This workout is the next step up for the intermediate exerciser or even for people who enjoy a challenge in their workout life.

Double workouts could be an option if you have 2 spaces over the course of a day so instead of one 50 minute session you could try two 25 minute bursts.

50 minute total body workout
30 minute challenge with intervals
2 minute sprints   2 minute press up challenge
2 minute sprint   2 minute squat thrusts
2 minute sprint   2 minute dynamic lunges
2 minute sprint   2 tricep dip or push up
2 minute jogging   2 fast hard punches
2 minute high knee runs   2 minute upper cut torso twists
2 minute strides   2 burpees
2 minute stride runs with elevated heels
10 minute core oblivion
2 minutes of plank hand switches or total plank jumps
2 minutes 45% angle oblique rotations from an elevated crunch position
2 minutes lower abdominal burn extended leg heel pushes to sky
2 minutes alternating crunches with arms and legs rotating
2 minutes side plank with extended high arm touching underside of body
10 minute yoga intense stretching-check out the best yoga classes and websites for total body moves-this is essential as every muscle has been pushed to the highest limit.

The next step after a few weeks of this programme is adaptation to exercise type and session time, boot camps should be introduced daily with two days of swimming added-if working out six days weekly try tackling the boot camp on Monday, Tuesday and Thursday with the Wednesday and Weekend day used for the swim session.

SWIMMING IDEAS

Swimming sessions sometimes can become boring for those who are used to gym work. Once you find your feet in the water and are assured of depth and ability try to progress from basic swim lengths up and down the pool to intervals with challenging movements.

INTERVALS

30 minutes of intervals can kick off with width sprints and recoveries. Do a sprint up and recovery crawl back until the 30 minute session is completed, now obviously this will become boring after a while so mix it up with swim strokes or add in a halfway challenge of double sprints or as many sprints as you can manage in 5 minutes.

Alternative challenge:-
If you want a change try adding in a total body challenge after 15 minutes. Swim to the pool side and roughly shoulder height water then perform the following:-

1. 40 consistent high knee movements with animated arms
2. 40 fast feet with exaggerated arm push movements
3. Hold onto side whilst lengthening body, switch on core and kick legs vigorously for a count of 20
4. 20 high knee jumps in water
5. Once this has been completed take a breath and get back into the remaining 15 minutes intervals. Remember to allow a 5 minute easy swim cool down and stretch in the water afterwards.

6. After 6 weeks of this session it is sensible to change the interval intensity and proceed to length ways swimming. In addition you could make your halfway mark more challenging with bigger bolder exercises-bounding and jumping in the water is easier especially if you have injuries.

TOP TIP

If you are feeling particularly energetic following your session you could empty your tank by timing yourself with length double swim (usually the time for swimming exams is 20\20 seconds up and down) over the block of six weeks you could endeavour to shave seconds off your time and prove that you are becoming more efficient in this type of training. Always think outside the box and use the pool to your advantage by creating new swimming sequences, exercises, challenges and strokes but be safe in whatever you attempt.

The Busy Professional Workout

Working long hours and having limited time for food breaks can play havoc with sugar levels and lead to weight gain. Long hours without snack stops leads to the human body dropping into survival state - leading to existing body fat being stored and energy levels plummeting. In order to maximize mental and physical well-being it is essential to feed your body at least every four hours.

FOOD

Fill any available cupboard at work with healthy snacks of choice and bottles of water. Graze through the day as you work at your desk or wherever you may be with oatcakes, nuts, fruit and seeds. Maintain important hydration levels with the water, remember that your brain needs carbohydrates to operate properly and your body needs water to fulfil every process properly.

WORKOUT

An office or workplace unit can become a multi gym if you use an active imagination. Jogging on the spot is easy anywhere, a sturdy chair helps with press ups, tricep dips, elevated lunges, and elevated planks.

Your star option would be to invest in a core ball and take it to work - at around ten pounds you have the perfect workout tool. Your core work can be done as you sit at your desk and at break time you can blast the fat with a pumping strength/cardio session.

WORKOUT PLAN

Always warm up prior to sessions with movements similar to the main component but with significantly less effort. Perform the moves until you feel loose mobility, warmer body temperature and a steady breathing pattern.

A super effective burst consists of:-
10 ELEVATED
10 SECONDS FAST PACE JOGS ON THE SPOT INTERSPERSED WITH 10 SECONDS BRIEF BREATHE BACK RESTS.
10 SQUATS OR SQUAT JUMPS IF YOU LIKE THE HEEL HYDRAULICS AND FEEL FIT ENOUGH.
10 PRESS UPS ON THE CHAIR OR CORE BALL
10 SCISSORS OR SHUFFLES WITH YOUR FAST FEET
10 ROCKY PUNCHES ON THE SPOT (the sound track usually helps me here)
10 SECONDS OF HIGH KNEE RUN ON THE SPOT BURSTS INTERSPERSED WITH BRIEF BREATHE BACK REST INTERVALS.
10 SECONDS OF PLANK HOLD WITH 10 SECONDS OF ALTERNATE ARM LIFTS OFF WITH THE OPPOSITE ARM FOR SUPPORT x 10.
10 STAR JUMPS OR JACKS

Remember that you can adapt any exercise to suit your fitness levels or preference if you have weak ankles or knees – a side step can easily replace a jack as long as you maintain effort with high exaggerated arms.

THE HOUSE WORK WORKOUT SESSION

No excuses! If you run a busy household and have a large family you will be tired and trying to fit time to exercise in. Help is here, if you are on the run the grazing idea will keep your food habits in check so all you need is the exercise.

Get ahead of the game before you even leave the house with household chores.

WORKOUT PLAN

Cleaning windows inside and out presents the perfect opportunity for muscle strength gains and improved flexibility.

Use a lower stool for windows - this will force you to engage your core to reach, switching on your stability muscles. Having to stretch that bit harder lengthens the working muscles and improves flexibility. Lifting and carrying the cleaning tools from the back door as oppose to the front door allows you to spend extra time weight training.

Hoovering is a very effective core and upper body strength exercise. By turning your hoover to a deep pile setting you will have to push harder to move it thus engaging core muscles you take for granted. Pushing that bit harder through the core and forcing change of direction with the shoulders and arms adds up to a dynamic upper body challenge. This movement is also true of pathway or drive sweeping, pushing against the force of the garden fodder you sweep allows the core to fire up. If done with vigour this utilises the cardio effort in the workout, combining in sessions saves loads of time and forces the body to work harder for short bursts melting away the fat stores.

The leg muscles gain from deep squats which are perfect when cleaning ovens, low cupboards or fridges, baths and under sinks - get into a deep squat position and start cleaning. Refresh the squat position every twenty seconds by shifting position from side to side or up and down slightly – to be honest though this will probably happen automatically as you shift your weight naturally.

Now for the final burst in this session – mattress flipping, this consists of core work, upper body strength, leg stability and cardio. Most people simply spread the duvet over the bed and go but this area is a dream for housework exercisers.

Flipping your mattress several times before making the bed will have you sweating and breathing heavy burning calories. Your whole body will be working spinning a double or king size padded weight like that.

THE NEW MUM WORKOUT
Young Mothers have the best equipment to work with in their quest to become a lean machine. A baby naturally progresses in weight and size which offers the Mother ready made strength work. Not only does breast feeding burn fat in new Mothers but as they are constantly on the move with the baby they can easily graze and burn extra calories on the go.
Performing abdominal exercises is not possible for Mothers until they have reached the stage where their abdominals have completely returned to the original state. Abdominal exercises are extremely dangerous when abdominals are split so take caution when checking your eligibility after child birth – always invest in a great Ante Natal manual. This rule applies to pregnant women also as lying on their back performing any exercise can place the Mother under strain in relation to the baby's position. A pregnancy activity manual will cover these factors as well as overhead weight lifting during pregnancy.

WORKOUT

12 BICEP CURLS WITH BABY

12 LUNGES FORWARD WITH BABY AT CHEST HEIGHT ON ALTERNATE LEGS.

12 SHOULDER PRESS WITH BABY HELD FIRMLY

12 CORE ROTATIONS HOLDING BABY AT TUMMY HEIGHT WITH PARTIALLY LENGTHENED ARMS.

12 BACK LUNGES WITH BABY AT CHEST HEIGHT ON ALTERNATE LEGS.

12 DEEP SQUATS HOLDING BABY AT SHOULDER LEVEL

12 FRONT RAISE WITH BABY BEING LIFTED TO THE FRONT WITH LENGTHENED ARMS AND STRONG FOREARMS AND SOFT ELBOWS.

12 EASY BABY SWINGS FROM ONE CORNER TO THE OPPOSITE OUTER THIGH (much like a wood chop) ALTERNATING ON BOTH SIDES.

BETWEEN EACH EXERCISE PERFORM 12 SIDE STEPS HOLDING THE BABY AT SHOULDER OR CHEST LEVEL.

Progressions in this case would be baby weight, exercise choice changes, increasing the repetitions on the least difficult exercises and also adding in short bursts of fast feet and running on the spot – ensuring that the baby is in a safe viewing place for this portion.

THE WORKOUT THAT WILL BURN FAT FASTER AND HEALTHIER

When deciding upon your exercise plan try to always perform strength work like weight training and kettle bell lifting before any type of free unrelated cardio like running, swimming, cycling and aerobics. When the muscles fire up in strength work the glycogen stores will be utilised, this means that your carbohydrate stores in the muscle will become the fuel source leaving your fat stores ready to go in the cardio section.......BOOM!

If you only have a short amount of time for a quick workout try combining cardio with strength. My boot camp sessions mix both and push the exerciser harder but for a shorter time, a sample consists of:-
PARK FAT GUZZLER SESSION
START WITH 10 JACKS OR STAR JUMPS
20 GRASS ALTERNATE THRUST
10 SPRINTS IN QUICK SUCCESSION TO THE NEAREST TREE
20 BOX OR FULL PRESS UPS
10 SCISSORS, SHUFFLES OR SPOTTY DOGS WITH EXTENDED ARMS
20 THRUST OR QUAT JUMPS
10 SRPINTS TO A TREE OR OBJECT AT LEAT TEN FEET FURTHER AWAY.
20 ALTERNATE ARM AND LEG PLANK HOLDS (count one for each appendage lifted from the grass)
10 BEAR WALKS IN SUCCESSION TO THE FURTHER AWAY TREE (you decide if you want to push yourself and count 10 up and down or 10 there and 10 back).
20 KNEE LIFT RUNS THE LENGTH OF AT LEAST 20 FEET AND BACK
FINISH WITH JOG, RUN OR SPRINT BACK HOME (combining 2 of the choices mentioned create effective interval training – i.e. 20 seconds sprint followed by 20 seconds jog all the way home).

Interval training is a saviour to many when it comes to burning fat and becoming a fit machine faster than they ever thought possible.

Intervals have become the choice of people who get bored easily in their sessions. Not only will interval training help you finish in half the time but it will keep you interested and working harder. It can be done in a pool or on land, on a bike or in the boxing arena, from aerobics to football every exerciser and athlete rely upon immense virtues of Intervals.

This type of training combines a burst of exercise for a short period of time with a rest period. It allows you to push yourself for that time knowing that you have a rest up ahead, alternately when you rest you become highly motivated to work even harder next time – it is a win, win situation.

The best news is that this technique taps into the energy system that utilizes fat for fuel, constant bursts mean constant taps into the fat source.

If u need any exercise description you can find it on any recognised health professional website or in a trusted fitness publication.

CHAPTER 14

ARNIE YOU AIN'T GIRL
LIFTING WEIGHTS

Cardio alone will not allow you to sculpt and define the strength and appearance of your physique. Lifting weights, kettle bells, power clubs or even body weight effectively strengthen areas of your body that you don't always take full advantage of. Lifting benefits movement, power, ability and agility. You'll prevent aches, pains, diminish stiffness and alleviate the ailments that come with standing, lying or sitting incorrectly.

Strengthening the muscles that support movement is important and helps as you get older. The bonus of course is that lifting helps to build a sculpted body to be proud of and the more lean muscle you possess the higher your ability to burn calories.

THE ULTIMATE FAT BURNER THAT HELPS EVERYONE

Pool work is understated to say the least and has a wide range of health benefits to not only the seasoned exerciser but to special populations. Swimming allows working muscles to push, pull, extend and contract. The ability to stay afloat whilst pushing against a dynamic force utilises the cardio vascular system to the max and calls on every muscle in the body to fire up, swimming daily for a few weeks can torch as much as 14 pounds of fat.

Aqua exercise is perfect for many different special populations, pregnant women, people with high blood pressure, cardiac patients, the obese, lower limb injury rehab people, arthritis sufferers and the elderly can all benefit from an aqua session.

Keeping the water just above core level will maintain a safe temperature, buoyancy of the water prevents weight loading, movement is gentle and injury risk minimal, flexibility improves and circulatory function also.

Health issues can be reduced and in some cases reversed with the help of simple pool work.

Groundhog Day exercise sessions
Keep everything fresh when you engage in your exercise routines, remember that like the mind the physique will never gain improvements by replicating the same routine. Shock the body with energetic additions of dance, martial arts, body weight exercises, swims and interval runs and only then will you see an athlete with a rocking body!

Adapting sessions to a higher level is something that should be easy to recognise. Enjoyment is quite obviously the most noticeable indicator of when to plan a change soon-when people know what to do and when they will start to enjoy other factors in the class such as music, I always think that once someone knows the words to a song it is time to change. I refer to timescale and boredom here, after a certain amount of time the body will need a greater challenge and the crowd will need to be kept on their toes as will the instructor. Around the six weeks mark there will be indicators to the aforementioned but the next step should be planned well before this point. Challenge is numero uno in this industry whether it be personal or professional, I often throw in some sessions that are alien to me like swimming or basketball drills to keep me fresh and hungry-there are times when we are thrown into alternative sessions due to injury or location-you certainly don't need a gym to train. I have to say that aqua training is beneficial to the performance of your preferred training plan. You'll enhance CV strength, explosive power, muscle strength and flexibility.

Since the 1980's it seems that a gym workout has been the preferred choice for most with the leg warmer craze becoming the most redeeming memory of what to expect in gyms-around 80% of exercisers aspired to this notion of the spandex physique with the other 25% striving to be themselves and choosing the pool or outdoors. The 25% have a lot to be proud of as they influenced the exercisers of Today to think outside the box and take to the great outdoors with kettle bells, power clubs and nature as tools. The spandex has been ditched for body armour and the people of Today are hard core and ready to take on any challenge from trees to dog chases.

It is so refreshing to see that the skinny has been overtaken by the strong! Health now prevails and image is a rewarding by product of it. The fitness industry has done a full 360 with men engaging in yoga and women flipping tyres, both sexes are realising that they have a lot to gain by exploring every area of health and fitness. Stereotypes still exist in gymnasiums everywhere but luckily the weight lifting poser who lifts nothing but his ego is being pushed aside by the human female ants lifting their own body weight. The females now couldn't care less about the sweaty dishevelled look as they know that their men prefer it and that is based on research carried out in 2010. Around half the gyms in Glasgow where the males (and in particular the males who train with partners) trained where bombarded with interviewers who questioned the response to women who took exercise seriously, engaged in many genres of fitness and left sessions looking 'well exercised'.   In conclusion to the questions 85% of men stated that they admired women who had actively participated in exercise to the detriment of their appearance and 75% of this group went on to say that they found this type of woman attractive with more likelihood of approaching them for a chat. Only 5% did not bother either way and 10% felt that this look was not particularly attractive, going on to say that their ideal women would resemble Paris Hilton and Katie Price.

In this day and age most of the population has taken note that exercise and health means a great deal more than a stroll on the treadmill or those uneventful crunches. The nation has embraced total body maintenance- more people want to learn more about improving health as well as body shape. Body images are far more positive these days thanks to the mega thigh media stars who serve as fantastic role models for the next generation of gym regulars.

CHAPTER 15

STRONG IS THE NEW SEXY

After the workouts done and the results start to appear it is gratifying to feel proud of a strong body. Gone are the days of stick thin models and pop stars as credible role models. Men admire and women aspire to a lean assured physique that would not look out of place in any sporting arena.

From dancing on ice to the most recent Olympics event there was great admiration when the female contenders unveiled their sculpted abdominals and unleashed thighs of stronger stuff then what women have been used to in recent years.

The Posh spice effect has been replaced by Jessica Ennis and Flavia Cacace.

Modern day men's attitude to women's figures now mirror that of the 50's 60's and 70's when females had functional physiques. The sort of women who looked like they could rear a dozen children whilst running a household and even changing all four car tyres single handed - perhaps even flipping a few!

Over 78% of British men prefer a fuller bottom and thighs with 80% favouring athletic looking arms and backs also.

Empowerment in the fitness stakes has become an aphrodisiac in this modern age which means good news for our children. In light of the horrific eating disorders of the 80's and 90's, it is comforting to know that the children of future years will be equipped with role models of stern stuff.

Aspiring to individual ideal of body image is the answer to a healthier existence as oppose to becoming influenced by the unattainable images of models and pop stars. This is an unachievable dream – creating one's own is far more rewarding.

There is sometimes an exception or two namely Pink, Beyonce, J-Lo and Rianna.

CHAPTER 16

EATING AFTER ALL EXERCISE SESSIONS

Following exercise of any type it is important to get nutrition right and follow any meal with an adequate drink.......not alcoholic!

Think of everything that the muscles have endured during the session. Glycogen (the energy that supplies the muscles during exercise ad in particular weight training) stores will be depleted so replenishing with adequate food choices is important not only for recovery but for the next session. Replenishing whilst affording rest through at least eight hours of sleep is the best remedy for punishing exercise sessions.

Without becoming too scientific in the description of glycogen it is important to know that when you intend to reduce weight that if you perform weight training prior to cardio exercise you will succeed in emptying glycogen stores during training with kettle bells, weights, power bags and body weight then burn fat as you perform any cardio from running to swim sprints.

Think ahead whenever you train and consider the next meal-quality carbohydrates, protein and good fats will take care of every need the body has. The muscle will benefit from the carbs and protein and joints exude with the help of quality omega rich fats. Refer to food choice chapters and reliable internet sources for more guidance.

When touching upon food and choices it is important to mention food diaries and the value they have in preventing present and future food choices. They have been used for years as a way of gathering and collating information about clients that whilst may seem unimportant to them can be invaluable for an instructor in gaging the moods that govern food choices.

Diaries are useful for the instructor to gain evidence but should be more so to the writer as this as useful a tool in weight loss as exercise itself. Completing ideas regarding session content and food choice in Ernest within the diary will prevent any short comings when it comes to executing what is on the agenda for every workout day.

This system can offer order in busy lives and combat situations that lead to reckless empty calorie consumption. It is amazing how a gym visit can fail because the recipient has lack of ideas or has failed to eat at the correct times in the day. Completing the diary the night before over a cup of tea will provide clarity of mind and a day that runs smoothly afterwards-you'll know exactly what you want to do and have the motivation to do it. It is truly amazing how these simple steps can replace doubt with self-belief. Think of the old double path adage that you see in films where there is good and evil and replace an unhealthy evening of rushed pizza and with an organised gym session and meal in front of the television with your work all done.

CHAPTER 17

TROUBLE SHOOTING YOUR WAY THROUGH THE MOST COMMON FAT BURNING CONSTRAINTS

Now that you have the knowledge to guide you confidently through a new life of eating enjoyable foods and exercising efficiently it is time to help yourself and others with personal experience.

Most people are caught napping at one point in their new life of greater health and this is totally normal. It does in fact benefit your will power and self-belief and teaches you that small bumps in the road will re-affirm your strength.

Recognising these barriers and embracing any weakness will help bolster your belief in yourself and life choice. These experiences will serve as good remedies for others to learn from also so share with fellow fat burners and exchange anicdotes.......no man is an island. By sharing experiences with others you as a group will find that no situation will be a challenge so here are some of the barriers I came up against whilst learning to reduce weight safely.

SCENARIO 1 THE CINEMA MUNCHIES
Most 'diet' gurus will tell you that you can enjoy cinema dates and still eat healthily.........no person who enjoys food wants to sit with a pack of rice cakes and water whilst everyone else is tucking into nachos and fizzy juice so compromise and enjoy the cinema experience.

A/Use your treat allowance and take whole grain snacks with a designated chocolate or alternative sweet treat. I find that taking my small flask of coffee helps me savour my treat as I have it with me and don't have to cue for one that will be cold when I finally get to my seat, the extra cup will also help to fill me up for the whole film.

B/I really do not like hotdogs or nachos so I tend to make my own little packed snack with my favourite humus and crackers or red peppers slices. Not only does my snack last longer but I feel like I'm actually savouring a small meal with the addition of cucumber batons. Sometimes I crave a warm option so I simply prepare a wholegrain baguette or pitta and place it in my food warmer bag which keeps it toasty for the film-these bags act like flasks and can also keep cucumber cool so check out choices online.

SCENARIO 2 CELEBRATIONS AND BIRTHDAY PARTIES

Birthday teas, Christenings and children's parties are all enjoyable events but can be a minefield of incorrect food choices for what you wish to gain. When I am faced with a plateful of sausage rolls or cocktail sausages I have the tendency to jump in, this is a common feeling among people who have problems controlling what they eat but with power of the mind and compromise you can still enjoy yourself. The treat saving option is perfect for these events (no one can possibly enjoy a party without the food and those who say otherwise must lead boring lives) this is a one off but be aware and listen to your bodies signals-back down when you receive the signal that you are full without discomfort. Always think back to how you felt when you shovelled the sausage rolls in...... bloated and fed up-I find that this usually works for me. Having an evening meal replaced by party food is not a mistake if you choose multi grain sandwiches and whole foods-in this day and age it is important that people cater for not just vegetarians but for the health conscious. Whenever I host I always choose the food wisely and have extra tasty whole grain snacks to which the junk food eaters devour without knowledge of how healthy they are eating. I prepare dark chocolate covered fruits and marsh mallows whilst I blend pure fruit juices for the cocktails-this is no more effort than preparing basic party foods and I can contribute to the health of my party goers too. When you have a couple of treats at the party try to have green or ginger T to help cleanse and by all means top up on water as this will help to aid digestion and fill you up. A decent size slice of cake can always replace the treat for the day and take it home with you to savour it at a time when you normally enjoy your treat. I find also that having grapes, nuts, seeds and whole grain crackers for a snack before an event can stave of hunger ideas and limit what I eat during. Carrying out these ideas just once will surprise you and before you have time to doubt your ability you'll be enjoying parties and reducing the stress you used to experience because of a small thing like food.

SCENARIO 3 NERVOUS BINGING

There are times when nervous nibbling can lead to bad food choices and irregular eating. Exams, job interviews, WRITING BOOKS and exciting events can lead to nervous eating. Mind-set is important but it does also help to be prepared by using the diary to plan food choices ahead, surrounding yourself with adequate food choices will help to ease your burden. Studying is usually done in slots so use bowls of warm nuts, whole grain crisps, homemade bran treats and fruit slices to keep you satisfied and feed your brain-these choices will also keep sugar levels stable.

SCENARIO 4 WINTER WARMING NOSH

During this time it is only human to seek warmth and satisfaction through food. In Britain the winter months tend to last half the year so this could make a big impact on the Nations weight. We are missing one important element at this time of year and that is that colder climates allow us to burn fat more efficiently. After heat seeking workouts we should choose the foods that not only satisfy us but are the most nutritious, I speak of whole foods such as nuts, oats, hearty vegetables and grains. IDEAS:-

-Cinnamon porridge is not only good for you it stabilizes sugar levels and creates energy when you need it.

-A baked apple with honey and ginger or cinnamon will act as a tasty treat and provide warmth.

-Brown pasta tossed in chopped nuts, red peppers, a small amount of olive oil and grated feta creates a warming tasty lunch with energy benefits.

-Couscous fluffed and mixed with chopped boiled eggs, flaked almonds, peppers and a drizzle of soya sauce is the ultimate feel good food.

Try all the dishes above and experiment with recipes before the winter months approach in order to prepare for the easy dishes you'll enjoy.

SCENARIO 5 EATING OUT

Dining out need not be a minefield so empower yourself with confidence when dining out and don't be afraid to ask your waiter to alter anything you wish to choose in order to make it suit your needs. If you order a meal and request something be taken out it'll mean that the restaurant wins saving money on that ingredient.

Drinks are easy to navigate around, the beer should be reduced gradually, cocktails can be altered with certain sugary ingredients being replaced with natural juices, wine can be enjoyed in moderation, try sipping water between each drink and with dinner to avoid dehydration.

CHAPTER 18

DRESSING FOR YOUR NEW BODY

Most people who lose weight and witness a remarkable change in their body shape almost certainly become overwhelmed with the whole prospect of what they perceive to be a 'new identity'- so much so that they find it hard to adjust and rely upon baggy clothes for a sense of comfort. This sense of comfort reassures you that 'you are still you' even though your body looks completely different.

Some successful weight reducers however tend to adopt a completely different approach and the weight loss takes over the personality they had before. They become a 'Hollywood' version of their former self (no disrespect to any Hollywood folks) and self-confidence almost translates into arrogance. I always take the opportunity to promote self-confidence because without it we are nothing but to lose your original identity in the hype of a new slender body is a fast track route to you falling flat on your ass.

A new body and improved self-awareness should serve to enhance you as the person you where before, to help you aim higher and go for the goals that you thought where once out of reach. By all means motivate on all fronts but hold onto the humble attitude you had before. A new frame means more than just a change of wardrobe it means aiming for a better job, a fitness goal or perhaps a new partner – your attitude to yourself will change but so will the attitude of others toward you, the only drawback to that for me was the wallies who wanted to speak to me once I had gained my slim self when before they probably laughed at my size with their intellectually challenged friends.

Body size reduction is just like obesity in that the person's psychological state becomes 50% of the problem, the personality of a heavy person is complex and prone to severe self- doubt episodes. The constant tugging of the jumper over the bum and tummy is one of the most annoying habits that I found myself displaying. Habits like these never fade even though I am now a size eight – once you see yourself as heavy the image sticks in your head and even after successful weight loss pops up now and again.

Many times I found myself looking in the mirror and scrutinizing the slim frame that other people saw. Although I could never see why Anorexic sufferers could get so thin without noticing it, I could understand to a small extent how mind set can be so stubborn that you develop a modified picture of yourself no matter what other people tell you. I knew that this habit of mine would never spiral out of control because 99% of the time I couldn't believe how much I had achieved when I looked in the mirror…….I was happily dumfounded.

Losing weight just takes some getting used to because effectively we are renting a whole new body – I say renting because body shape can change at any time, keeping up the rental requirements is important to future slender success :-

1. Look in the mirror daily and remind yourself of the amazing journey you have personally achieved so far and how many friends you have inspired.

2. Keep a picture of your former self in your bag so that you carry a wee boost around with you for times when you need it. This also helps when people don't believe how fantastic you are as it provides proof.

3. Save all the money you would have spent on bad habits and when you enough spend it fortnightly or monthly on a show stopping piece of clothing, not only will you appreciate checking yourself out in those multiple changing room mirrors

but you'll boost your confidence with a sexy little number that highlights your new physique.

4. If you have a face book to twitter account use it for a positive reason and inspire others by logging your new lifestyle, include healthy food tips that helped you or some positive slimming ideas that just might influence more people than you think to take the step to engage in better eating.

5. Break out and attempt bigger goals in your career or personal endeavours. You'll succeed and remind yourself how far you really have come – set those success goals.

6. Keep the fire in your belly burning by setting up a club which inspires others to lose weight in a healthy way – share all the secrets that helped you and observe whilst others succeed, this provides a great deal of pride for you and your group believe me. Take that next step to learn more about the back ground of nutrition and health by enrolling in a course or degree – it is beneficial for you when you have the scientific picture of how the human body actually operates and transfers energy. Educational understanding of this field will keep you safe in the knowledge that you have more to teach people and there is a staggering amount of slimmers who took the step to swap their chosen career for nutrion or fitness careers simply because they were so inspired by their journey – let's face it we are all walking proof of what we teach so what more could people who learn from us ask for.

CHAPTER 19

THE MOTIVATION TO KEEP MOVING FORWARD

Anytime a person successfully reduces weight there are more benefits than just the personal opinion they have of themselves. Motivation comes in the shape of shopping in shops that they once rushed past because of the self-loathing they felt – especially the under wear shops that slim girls take for granted. However it also comes in the kind words of other people – observations of other people is a powerful tool in motivating a slimmer as these opinions are usually voluntary and 100% honest which provides a tangible reality to the achievements of the slimmer.

In terms of physical feedback the new improved body has a new found energy pool that will make you feel invincible! Energy levels would have been as flat as your new tummy before the journey to lose weight started and the bi products of high energy levels are definitely the rushes of euphoria that you will experience when you can swim, run or sprint faster than you ever imagined. New foods and less weight to carry around provide these bursts of energy – do not under estimate how amazing you will feel daily. Maintaining the physique you currently enjoy will not be a problem as you will feel compelled to participate in new activities with family and friends...... your kids will love you for this because you really won't mind 'running amuck' in the park and acting like a big kid because you have a figure to envy.

The new attitude you have will ultimately enhance your social life as you will be encouraged to join new clubs, classes and even the gym where you will meet likeminded people who enjoy the new activities that you do. Mutual motivation will prevail as you bounce off your new fitness buddies. Once people immerse themselves in the joys of weight loss and related bonuses they open up to a whole new world of opportunities. This is always enough to compel them to move onward to an enriched life. Quick fix diets fail on so many levels because commitment to healthy weight loss is more than just eating food or drinking shakes in some cases. The ultimate healthy weight loss plan addresses everything from eating and mind set to dressing and future endeavours. This book is a comprehensive guide to everything that will arise when you start your journey to better health – every little step along the way you have answers and suggestions that will get you through any barrier successfully.......empathy is a great tool. The food choices suggested are compatible with the choices that people make in everyday life but with minor tweaks that taste even better. No unrealistic promises are made because I am confident that I can predict exactly how the participant of the plan will feel within the first day, week and month of the new improved lifestyle. I know that the plan speaks for itself and I never instruct radical changes in the lives of these people, nor do I ask them to deprive themselves. Most importantly I know how people engaged in the plan will think feel and act on any given day because I have been there and done that ....I have an answer for just about everything.

CHAPTER 20

FINAL THOUGHT FROM ME TO YOU

This is an on-going commitment with endless benefits.

Most people fall at the last hurdle because they assume that when their weight is off that they can fall into old habits. The saviour in cases like these is that habit takes over, your stomach becomes accustomed to small amounts and binges ultimately leave you feeling sick.......another trial and error for myself. I was under the impression that I could eat whatever I liked when I became slim but I found out that I no longer had a taste for binging on rubbish and if I overate at all I would feel like an upside down turtle.

I started to appreciate my treats and if I did overdo it I learned to not be as hard on myself and work off some of the offending foods in the gym. A balance can be struck as long as you moderate the treats you enjoy so inevitably you can stay slim whilst enjoying life.

This area is the most reason why I disagree with wonder diets and supplements. Most followers punish themselves for months drinking shakes and eating fat free foods (high sugar I might add) just to obtain 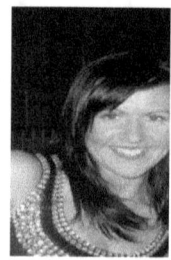 an ideal weight then start binging on the foods they miss when they achieve their ideal weight. I believe that if you can lose weight whilst enjoying the foods you like in moderation and with compromises then you will never feel the need to binge. Living this way will leave you never having to dread the feeling of a Monday morning again.

Love and warm wishes
Michelle